The Sexu

Exploring the Realities of Human Sexuality

By Grace Ennis

Table of Contents

Introduction 4

Chapter 1: Understanding the Psychology of Sexuality 8

Chapter 2: Society and Sexual Freedom 14

Chapter 3: Double Standards and Sexual Expression 21

Chapter 4: Issues Related to Sexuality 26

Chapter 5: How Sexuality is Addressed in Therapy 32

Chapter 6: The Sexualization of Women 39

Chapter 7: Sexual Violence Against Women 48

Chapter 8: Sexual Expression Through Pornography 54

Chapter 9: Addicted to Pornography 67

Chapter 10: When Sexual Expression Breaks Down Marriages 77

Chapter 11: The Religious View of Sexual Expression 86

Conclusion 108

Introduction

Why is it that society is so misinformed about human sexuality? If you spend some time analyzing how the world we live in views sex you will come to a very quick conclusion! It isn't something that's spoken about, instead sex education has been reduced to subliminal messages from the media that have done and continue to do more harm than good. Where do we get our knowledge about human sexuality? Are the sources reliable and trustworthy? What reference point are we using to determine whether what we see and hear from media outlets is the truth?

The majority of parents leave sex education to the school because they don't understand it themselves. However, how many hours can the average student say they have spent in a class about human sexuality? The answer is going to be not many because it's not a subject that people want to talk about when it should be one of the most important discussions we are having in our society. It's easy to point out a flaw when you have knowledge about a subject that is presented to you, however, when you are ignorant about the topic, you have nothing to base your information against.

We are not talking about sexuality, but 40 million people in America are secretly watching pornography online. If the only sexual education we are getting is coming from pornography, we are missing the spiritual and emotional components of sexual intimacy.

In some cultures it's considered inappropriate to openly talk about human sexuality or the human body in general. This can make it very difficult to educate a teen about sexuality.

There appears to be a misconception that if sex is not spoken about then our teenagers won't practice it. Limiting sexual education and pushing the abstinence agenda without explaining why can actually encourage sexual risk taking and increase unwanted pregnancy. If the youth are incapable of understanding human reproduction it only makes sense that avoiding it is going to be difficult. These avoidance strategies also lead to teenagers believing that they don't feel comfortable talking to their parents, teachers or other adults about sex and so they turn to their friends who are just as ignorant as they are.

Unfortunately sexual abuse, sexual harassment, and child abuse are a massive problem around the globe, could this be due to a lack of understanding about human sexuality? It's a discussion worth having; however, in this book you will learn about the psychology of sexual expression and the role that our culture has played in shaping it.

Chapter 1: Understanding the Psychology of Sexuality

Sexuality refers to an individual's preferences and habits in relation to sexual desire and behavior. There are so many individual sexual expressions that it is impossible to number them. Some people can become distressed or confused about their desired sexual behavior or their actual sexual behavior and get help from a therapist who has been trained to assist people in working through such issues. With professional help, individuals are capable of going on to engage in fulfilling and satisfying sexual relationships.

Human Sexuality

The idea of sexuality is personal and complex and involves more than just sexual activity. The majority of people have their own definition of sexuality. It may include their personal and moral values, how they feel about body image, the way they are intimate with others, and their attraction and feelings towards the opposite or same sex. Sexual expression can manifest through a variety of different ways including relationships, societal roles, behaviors, fantasies and thoughts. Despite the fact that a person's sexuality can be influenced by their gender, identity and orientation, they are all distinct concepts. The sex of an individual is based on the sex that was given at birth based on their physical features. While gender identity is based on how a person feels internally about being male or female. Sexuality is not the same as sexual orientation; this refers to the individual experience of sexual attraction.

Sexuality is also seen as a developmental process because it can evolve and change over time. A child learns about intimacy and love from their primary caregivers. Children are known to participate in sexual play while playing games such as doctor between the ages of 4 and 8. When adolescents start to experience puberty they may begin to experiment with masturbation and other mild forms of sexual activity. An individual's sexuality continues to develop as they enter into young adulthood. In many cultures at this stage it is common for young adults to start thinking about a long term relationship. The desire for sex typically declines in old age although there is still the desire for intimate physical contact.

Culture and Sexuality

Culture is the main influence on sexuality; some researchers believe that environment plays a bigger role in determining a person's sexuality than genetics. What is considered the norm differs between religion, culture and historical periods. Norms and values differ between societies and in some cases the laws may differ. For example in some countries it's illegal to be homosexual.

From a young age people are taught whether directly or indirectly about the sexual norms of their culture. Ideologies are ingrained through the media, religious teaching and education classes. The most prevalent views related to sexuality in all societies are largely influenced by history, philosophy, religion and various other factors. In America, religion has played a major role in sexuality; however, over the years the media has promoted conflicting viewpoints regarding what is considered as sexually acceptable.

Despite the fact that there is no one culture that has the right view about sexuality, problems emerge when there is a conflict between individual sexuality and their cultural norms. For example, homosexual people often feel alienated from society because it is still considered unacceptable in some parts of the world. In such cases, individuals experience an internal conflict over whether or not they should conform to the norms of the society or follow their own desires regardless of the persecution they may face. This struggle can lead to people living a double life where a man can have a wife and a family and have a secret boyfriend to fulfill their hidden desires.

Chapter 2: Society and Sexual Freedom

Actor Kristen Stewart has her picture taken at Cannes with her ex-girlfriend Alicia Cargile. Amandla Stenberg, the seventeen year old Hunger Games actor describes how hurtful it has been to fight for her identity when you are black, bisexual and female. The singer St Vincent sits on the front row of the London Fashion week and kisses her girlfriend Supermodel Cara Delevingne. Actor, DJ and model Ruby Rose describes herself as "extremely gender fluid," she added to this statement that as each day passes she feels more gender neutral.

Thirty years ago these stories would have received a massive amount of criticism. There is an even higher possibility that they would never have made it into the media in the first place. Today, it appears to be the norm for people to make public declarations about their sexuality. This is even more visible within the millennial generation. A survey published in the Archives of Sexual Behavior reported that there is an increase in people reporting that they are in same sex relationships, and there has been an increase in tolerance for these types of courtships.

It is clear that the younger generation are comfortable with gender fluidity, bisexuality, same sex relationships and many other lifestyles that fall outside of the norms of traditional living. According to journalist Laurie Penny who identifies as genderqueer and bisexual states that society's acceptance of diverse sexualities is do to the advances in technology. The internet has opened the door for people whose lifestyles do not fit the norms and values of the society that we live in. It gives them the opportunity to present themselves as human beings and not rebellious aliens who refuse to conform. Penny also goes on to state that a large number of celebrities who are either in a same sex relationship or they are open about discussing their gender in non-binary terms is causing a shift in the attitude. People like Ruby Rose and Miley Cyrus are giving other people the confidence they need to speak openly about their sexuality.

Political blog editor Niamh Ni Mhaoileoin, who describes herself as queer, is confident that the more famous and well known people live their non conventional relationships in front of the cameras, the more acceptable it will become and the quicker it will change. She believes that they are sending a positive message that being gay is only a part of your life and it doesn't dominate it.

Homosexuality is now a part of the political arena, Tory leader for Scotland Ruth Davidson is openly gay, she announced the proposal to her girlfriend Kezia Dugdale who is the Scottish Labor Leader publicly. Everyone appeared to be happy for them, when they both turned up as a couple to the polling station no one looked at them twice.

Ni Mhaoileoin says that she is overwhelmed by how drastically sexual perception is changing. When she announced that she was gay in 2008, she was severely victimized for her choice. When her and her girlfriend walked down the streets of Dublin, they had abuse hurled at them. She is glad to say that this is no longer the case. Her experience is that young people are more accepting of sexuality that isn't heterosexual. Older people will question her about why she was once in a relationship with a man but is now with a woman, where as younger people just accept it.

There are still parts of society that are not in agreement with non traditional relationships. Pat McCrory the governor for North Carolina signed a bill that banned transgender people from using bathrooms outside of the sex that they were given at birth.

Penny states that the situation is not as simple as we think. Yes people are becoming more accepting and tolerant but there is still a lot of prejudice and violence against people who refuse to conform to a gender, transsexual and queer people. Although certain strides have been made, it still isn't easy.

There is also discrimination within the gay community at large where bisexuals feel as if they are not accepted because they have had relationships with the opposite sex which means they didn't come out of the womb gay. Many bisexuals claim that they don't feel as if they are a part of the LGBTA community and the very nature of their sexuality excludes them from it.

This is the nature of sexual freedom, being able to define yourself on your own terms without feeling the need to explain yourself to anyone. Although tolerance is growing for non-heterosexual relationships there are always going to people who don't agree with it. If you have defined yourself based on the sexual liberty that we have your goal shouldn't be to get others to accept you, it should be to accept yourself.

Chapter 3: Double Standards and Sexual Expression

It appears that there always has been, and there always will be a double standard when it comes to male and female sexual expression. We all know the story, a man can sleep with 25 women in a week and get called a stud, but if a woman does it she is called all manner of derogatory names.

The media is largely responsible for constructing our expressions of sexuality. In film, on TV, and music. R&B and hip hop has played a large role in the degradation of the female. Jay-Z is one of the most famous rappers of our generation, he has a song called "I've got 99 problems but a bitch ain't one."

The images that we are exposed to through media outlets have an effect on the way we treat each other. Negative images about women and sexuality have an effect on the way men view and treat women.

The term "pimp" has been glamorized within popular culture, but if you are to study the origins of this word the meaning is far from glamorous. The word basically means a man who arranges paid sexual interaction between a client and a prostitute. The verb "to pimp" means a variation of the following: to exploit, dress up elegantly, dressing seductively. According to the Oxford Dictionary the word "pimp" means "a despicable person."

Despite the disturbing and negative history behind the word "pimp" it has adopted a positive and desired social meaning. There are men who actually take pride in being labeled as a "pimp" because today it means a man who lives a lavish and impressive lifestyle and has a string of different women.

The opposite is true of the adjectives that are used to describe women who work for the pimps. They are referred to as "whores," "sluts," and "bitches." These words have become socially acceptable, even to the point where that is how some women describe themselves.

The media has trained women to use their physical attractiveness to attract men. There is no emphasis placed on the intelligence, honesty and the integrity of a woman. Men on the other hand have been trained that their looks are largely unimportant. According to the media women are looking for men with power, money and status as potential partner. An unattractive women is not viewed as important in society, a man with no money is viewed in the same way. However, it is more realistic for a man to acquire wealth than for a woman to change her genetic makeup regardless of how much plastic surgery she may have.

Relationship expert and author Laura Brotherson coined the term "The Good Girl Syndrome," it is an explanation of the phenomenon where young girls are told that it is a dirty transgression to enjoy sexual acts. A young lady can be raised in an environment where sex has been such a strict and taboo subject that when she gets into a committed and stable relationship she can't forget what she has been taught to believe. This then makes it difficult for her to function in a sexual relationship. Instead of being taught sex is healthy in the right context, adult's present sex to youths in a negative way that can affect them in the future.

Young boys seem to learn about sex through the media and friends. Since we are living in an era where hyper sexualization is the norm and where society embraces male sexual expression and sexuality through masturbation, pornography, the objectification of women and casual sexual partners, we now have a generation of men who have been sexually empowered. Men who have received their sex education through the media and a generation of women who are confused about who they are supposed to be sexually.

Chapter 4: Issues Related to Sexuality

Sexual intimacy is supposed to be one of the most fulfilling and satisfying of all human physical experiences. However, for some people sexual activity is far from pleasurable. Issues related to sexual intimacy are often as a result of traumatic experiences that prevent an individual from being able to engage themselves fully in sexual pleasure. Therapist Jill Denton states that "Every individual has their own unique idea of sexuality that is partially formed through religious influences, the media, culture, childhood neglect or abuse and family. Some of these messages can have a negative effect on the healthy development of an individual's sexuality."

Sexual problems are also related to mental health issues such as anxiety or depression. Or they can be related to physical conditions such as childbirth, menopause, a change in hormone levels, medication, chemical imbalances, urinary or bowel problems. Sexual problems are very common, in America depending upon gender and age. There are an estimated 30 to 40 percent of people suffering from a sexual issue in the United States. For the individuals who seek therapy, the most common concerns include:

- Promiscuity
- Sexual compulsions or impulsions that cause distress
- Problems with body image
- Loneliness
- Recovery from sexual assault or abuse

- A conflict of sexual desire between couples

- Uncertainty or anxiety about sexual orientation

- A lack of sexual desire

- Impotence

- Sexual anxiety

The DSM manual (the manual that officially records mental disorders lists four diagnosable sexual disorders for men and three for women. There has been a lot of criticism related to the gender specific categorizations of sexual disorders. Recent studies have found that sexual interest/arousal disorder is not exclusive to females; it has also been recommended that a gender neutral category is included.

Male Sexual Disorders

- Premature ejaculation

- Erectile dysfunction

- Delayed ejaculation

- Hypoactive sexual desire

The DSM also lists several paraphilias which are the sexual preference for abnormal behaviors. They are listed as being a potential problem when certain criteria has been met. A paraphilia qualifies as a disorder when a non-consenting individual is harmed because of it or when an individual experiences psychological distress because of it. When a paraphilia is acted upon by two consenting adults it is not considered as a mental disorder. The following parahilias are listed in the DSM:

- Voyeurism

- Exhibitionism

- Transvestism

- Sexual sadism

- Sexual masochism

- Pedophilia

- Frotteurism

- Fetishism

The fantasies that are associated with such behaviors are generally not a cause for concern unless the person who is experiencing the fantasy is distressed by them. In fact the majority of these behaviors, bar pedophilia can be explored in a safe and healthy way between consenting adults. It only becomes a problem when individuals are harmed physically or psychologically by the act.

Chapter 5: How Sexuality is Addressed in Therapy

There are people who have no desire for sex and they are fine with it. There are others who become deeply distressed as a result of sexual issues. When an individual feels that their sexual questions or concerns may be viewed as inappropriate by friends, family and partners they can experience frustration and anxiety or even shame. These feelings then lead to further distress which can require therapy to resolve. Finding the right therapist often provides the individual with a safe environment where they discuss their sexual desires, memories, fears, fantasies or difficulties.

Sex therapists have been trained to help people who are struggling with sexual issues. They help individuals to remove or reduce emotional barriers that are preventing people from having satisfying sexual experiences. They treat people who have issues related to the following:

- Arousal and desire
- Performance
- Satisfaction
- Sexual abuse/trauma
- Pain during sex
- Confusion or conflict between sexual orientation

A variation of interventions are used during therapy such as:

- Identifying different forms of sexual expression

- Exploring the negative views that prevent sexual satisfaction

- Basic sex education

- Mindfulness practice to assist people in becoming present mentally during sex

- Exploring sexual fantasies

Regardless of whether the sexual problems are physical or emotional, a sex therapist is able to help people identify the psychological source of the problem. By treating the individual as a whole, physically and psychologically sex therapists have been successful in helping people to achieve sexual freedom. Here are some real life examples:

Anxiety About Sex Because of Childhood Experiences

A 48 year old man named Sam has been experiencing feelings of depression and anxiety. This has led to him turning to alcohol to cope with his feelings. Realizing that his problem was spiraling out of control he made the decision to go and see a therapist. During one of his sessions he reveals that he has never been in a long term relationship although he would like to have one. He has a number of casual relationships that ended in disaster when it came time to become intimate. Questions about what Sam desires romantically seemed to cause him some embarrassment. When the therapist made further enquiries Sam revealed that he felt shame about having sexual feelings. During his sessions he was able to address his feelings and it became apparent that they were related to his strict religious upbringing and a traumatic childhood experience of witnessing a teacher molest a young boy. Sam reported the incident, but he never received any counseling to help him cope with what he saw.

Now that he is able to do work through what he experienced and overcome the shame and fear, he is slowly starting to accept that his sexual desires are a healthy and normal part of life. He also overcomes his depression and anxiety, his social life is renewed and he can date with excitement, confidence and a positive outlook.

Understanding Sexual Attraction

Maria is 36 years old, and she has started to realize that she is attracted to women. Maria wants to talk about the way she is feeling with a therapist so that she can learn to understand them better. She reveals that she is happily married to her husband and she has no plans of divorcing him. However, she often feels overwhelmed, anxious, confused, excited and guilty about the feelings that she has for other women. She also reveals that she has been fantasising about a woman at work and she feels that the woman might also have the same feelings towards her. Maria isn't sure whether or not she should ignore how she is feeling or tell her husband. Therapy helps Maria to examine how she feels and the choices that she can make. They also talk about the best way she can communicate what she is experiencing with her husband.

In a later session Maria reveals that she has told her husband and that he is supportive of whatever she decides to do. She reported that he wasn't judgmental and his only requirement was that she continued to be honest in their marriage. Though Maria has yet to decide how she intends on pursuing the relationship with her co-worker or other possible partners she believes that her openness bought a new level of intimacy to her relationship with her husband. She expresses peace and confidence that the attraction she has to other women is a part of her nature and she also feels happy that she is still accepted and loved by her husband.

Chapter 6: The Sexualization of Women

In the Woman More magazine there was an article written by a psychotherapist named Anina Bena who describes how she made the decision to drive across the street from her office to go to lunch. Her reason for this was she was trying to avoid the catcalls she was forced to endure anytime she walked in that particular direction. The last time she crossed that street a middle aged man leaned out of his truck and shouted "Ride my dick baby!" She wondered how it would feel not to feel as if she was some kind of sexual object on display. She also thought about whether she would rather be the woman who gets male attention or the woman who doesn't.

In her profession Anina meets hundreds of women who struggle with their sexuality or body image. These struggles manifest through the following:

- Relationship crises

- Parenting issues

- Reproductive concerns

- Obsessive compulsive disorders

- Body dismorphic disorders

- Eating disorders

- Anxiety

- Depression

Anina also mentioned that she is seeing an increase in the number of men coming for therapy who are struggling with loneliness and other relationship issues, she goes on to discuss how she has had firsthand experience of not fitting into the social construction of beauty that the media bombards us with. As a Middle Eastern American she didn't fit the European ideal of beauty. When she was a young girl, all the pictures she drew were of blond hair blue eyed princesses. She also had a blonde stepsister to contend with who would confirm her insecurities and tell her that her skin was the same color as poop. No matter how hard she tried she was never going to be white.

Now that Anina has a full understanding of how normal body struggles are she has started to wonder who really has the problem, her clients or our culture? We are continuously bombarded with hyper sexualized images of women, so much so that society has become desensitized to them.

These images are everywhere, and because of the level of exposure, it has become normal to objectify females.

With the rapid advances in technology, the quality and quantity of these images have intensified. In the United States the online pornography industry generates $13 billion per year and generates $100 billion worldwide. This is bigger business than baseball, basketball and professional football combined. Researchers analyzed more than 1000 Rolling Stone covers published over the past 40 years and found that in the 1960's 44 percent of the women were portrayed sexually. In the 2000s, 83 percent of women were portrayed sexually.

The "breastaurant," chain are establishments where young attractive women serve in revealing uniforms are also on the increase. According to an article written by journalist Jillian Berman in 2015, breasturants have doubled in sales over the past year.

More young people are being exposed to sexual imagery. In a 2010 study conducted in the United Kingdom it was found that a third of 14 to 16 year olds had been exposed to sexual images on the internet when they were 10 years old or younger.

Social learning theory states that audiences can be persuaded to purchase a product if advertising narrative is frequently repeated and easily recognizable. If the majority of adverts contain images of women as sex objects what is this saying about the health of our society and how is it affecting those who are exposed to it?

Everyone is has fallen victim to the obsession with physical appearance. It encourages people to separate the individual person from the body since the main focus is on how they look. Every woman is affected regardless of whether or not they fit the conventional standards of beauty and whether the images that we are exposed to portray women as passive or active. This has reduced the body to an object that exists only for sexual pleasure which leads to self objectification. This then leads to sexual dysfunction, depression and eating disorders.

Studies have also found that there is a link between pornography and sexual violence. The continuous exposure of women as sex objects might encourage men to believe that they have the right to force women into sexual acts. Men also suffer physically and emotionally from being exposed to hyper sexualized images because they are also portrayed as over sexed beasts who are less than human. In her research psychologist Linda Musses found that husbands who often use pornography experience poor relationship quality and marital adjustment problems. Men as early as the age of 20 are also experiencing erectile dysfunction problems because they have been desensitized to sexual images.

Pornography has led a lot of men to become emotionally confused. On the one hand they crave real human connections but at the same time they are being taught to fulfill this need in unfulfilling and empty ways.

It seems like there is no end in sight and that the human race is living in a constant cycle of dysfunction. Is there any way to fix this mess? The first step is to make people aware that what is going on isn't normal. As a society we have to be brave enough to analyze what we are being exposed to and then be brave enough to challenge what society has attempted to convince us is acceptable and normal. We can see that there have been efforts made in this direction with movements such as the Dove Campaign for Real Beauty which displays realistic body types in advertisements and sponsors projects that are focused on improving the self esteem of women. The woman's underwear company Dear Kate rejects airbrushing and idealized models. The Always Like a Girl Campaign promotes female empowerment. These are companies that are selling and promoting products but they have chosen not to use sexualized images of women to do so.

Unfortunately, these establishments are definitely an exception to the rule. However, we can be hopeful in the fact that there are groups of people who are actively fighting against the sexualization of women by the media. There is a lot of new research in this area and it is promising. A study conducted by Ohio State University found that people had a more favorable view of brands that did not rely on sexuality to sell their products. It is clear that it is more than possible to treat people with respect and dignity at the same time as selling products. Maybe the true desire of the human race is to live in a cultural environment where we can all feel authentic and safe.

Chapter 7: Sexual Violence Against Women

Every year there is a two week convention at the United Nations headquarters to address the issues that are having the most affect on girls and women. In March 2016, the topic was centered around how the objectification of females in the media is connected to violence against girls and women.

An estimated 60,000 teenage girls are murdered every year. Out of 120 million young girls, one in ten of them have been victims of forced sexual acts or rape. In America, approximately 11 percent of high school girls have reported that they have been raped. According to the Violence Against Women Survey one in four girls have been subjected to sexual violence before the age of 18, and approximately one in four girls lost their virginity through forced sex. The question is why is violence against females so prevalent?

The American Psychological Association published a report in 2010 on female sexualization in the media. It discussed how the media exposes young boys to sexualized images of women teaching them that females are objects. Analyzing various media outlets, the study confirmed that girls are consistently portrayed as sexual objects in comparison to their male counterparts. They are scantily dressed, and their body language and facial expressions imply that they are available sexually. In a 2008 study conducted by researchers at Wesleyan University it was found that out of the 58 magazines evaluated, 51.8 percent of all advertisements displayed women as sex objects. They also found that magazines specifically tailored towards men portrayed women as sex objects 76 percent of the time.

The hyper sexualization of femininity that is continuously perpetuated by the media has negative effect on the physical, emotional and mental well being of young girls and women on a global scale. Consequences include:

- Depression
- Low self-esteem
- Eating disorders
- Feelings of shame
- Appearance related anxiety

According to the Self Esteem Dove Project only 11 percent of girls worldwide define themselves as beautiful. Six in ten girls shy away from participating in certain activities because they are so concerned about the way they look. In Japan, one in three six year olds have a negative body image. Australian girls report that one of their top three life worries is their body image. In the United States 81 percent of 10 year old girls are scared to put on weight. In 2009, over 110,000 girls in Brazil had reconstructive surgery.

These stereotypes do not only have a negative effect on girls, they also affect boys. The media teaches men that attractiveness and success are tied to aggression, dominance and power.

Advertisements set the yardstick for what a culture considers normal. When the media bombards us with power dynamics that harm and degrade women and imply that violence against them is trivial it reduces the probability that acts of violence, and in particular sexual acts of violence will be reported.

In 2000, the United States Department of Justice conducted a study on college women and sexual victimization. Researchers discovered that less than five percent of rapes were reported to the police. When asked for their reasons why, the most common reason stated by the rape victims was that they feared that they would not be taken seriously. This is a serious issue because when it comes to sex trafficking, rape on campus, domestic violence and date rape the only way for victims to get help is if they report what has happened to them. The authorities are powerless to help women who have been abused if they are not made aware that it is taking place. Therefore, it is the responsibility of our culture and media outlets to encourage women to report any offense regardless of how small, an attack should be seen as harmful, serious and unacceptable.

Unfortunately, the media is doing nothing to empower women. Instead they send messages to females that state they need be beautiful and not bold; seen and not respected. These messages are not only harmful to women, young girls and their development, but to our culture in general.

Chapter 8: Sexual Expression Through Pornography

Some time ago I read a magazine article by a woman who had labeled herself as a feminist. She made claims that she enjoyed having sex with different men and that she didn't feel the need to be in a relationship with them to do so. In the same article she shared her disappointment that the men she slept with were not interested in her as a person, their desire was for her to act like a porn star and fulfill their fantasies. She felt as if she was being used to do nothing else than to satisfy a mans desire to indulge in the pornographic images he had exposed himself to. She complained that they were not tender, they had no desire for intimacy and there was definitely no love involved. Her body was being used for their pleasure and nothing else. She was horrified by what she was experiencing but at the same time she felt that her feminist standpoint gave her no room to explain her disgust and discomfort. After all, if she claimed that she was having sex with random men because she enjoyed it, why should she expect her partners to treat her like a romantic partner? People will treat you the way you treat yourself and if you have made yourself available for no strings attached sex don't complain when you get just that.

We are living in a generation where men are drowning in a cesspool of pornography and this has produced new expectations for what they desire from a woman. They want the women they sleep with to disregard their true nature and act like a porn star which leaves women feeling used and in some cases lower then a prostitute, at least they get paid to act like that.

At the touch of a button whether on a cell phone or a laptop sexual stimuli is available on demand. The easy access to a variety of images means that people are able to look at whatever they want and look at it whenever they want. In doing so they can serve, satisfy and generate their sensual nature. Pornography has created a world where the consumer (typically men) has the ability to access graphic images of sexual encounters and nudity. Women are available for their pleasure when they want, there are no immediate consequences and people become disposable objects.

The debate about the positives and negatives of pornography is taking place on blogs, websites, the news, television, in the pulpits and in government institutions. There are voices on every side of the conversation, sociologists, First Amendment advocates, feminists, theologians, atheists, conservatives and liberals and those who are against it are all shouting one unanimous message. Pornography is turning the nation into emotionless, sex obsessed beasts, and there doesn't appear to be an end in sight.

Pornography has turned sex into a consumable product. Those watching it begin to view human beings as objects that they can buy as opposed to individuals who are deserving of dignity. Sex is taken out of its proper context when it is consumed for the benefit of another person.

Searching for a picture, website, video or magazine with the right image to give you what you need provides the promise of connection and euphoria.

In their book SuperFreakonomics Stephen Dubner and Steven Levitt dedicated an entire chapter to investigating the economy of prostitution. They detailed several interesting findings; the taboo sexual acts that demanded a premium price years ago are now considered the norm. What was formally forbidden has now become mainstream which has lowered the price of the acts significantly. Sex acts that were once taboo because of their degrading and vile nature are now accepted as normal forms of sexual expression in a relationship. Normal sex is now considered undesirable and boring; the new normal is now degrading and invasive.

Pornography is inherently unloving and violent it has perverted the true nature of sexuality and teaches that degradation and violence for the purpose of pleasure is normal. It has reduced sex to the immediate gratification of an individual's most base desires. It exists beyond morality, ethics and rules and yet it is impossible to number the amount of men who are getting married and bringing their baggage of pornography with them. Having been exposed to thousands of unnatural sex acts they then load these expectations on their wives. The husband demands that his wife is willing to do what he wants and she is expected to be just as skilled and eager as the women who he has seen on screen.

Having surrendered themselves to a debased nature of pornography men have had their entire perception of sexuality shaped and altered by professional actors. They then impose these impossible expectations of a porn star onto their wives and this is where the trouble begins. There are definitely a combination of reasons why men cheat on their wives or partners, but one of them is that they don't feel as if their sexual needs are being met. The sexual needs that have been formed from years of addiction to pornography. According to statistics, approximately 40 million people in America watch online pornography on a regular basis. Pornography is a worldwide economic industry with the human body as its product. The production process includes links to drugs, prostitution, child pornography, human trafficking and other forms of violence. Economically it feeds mainstream industries, and these include Wall Street, media production companies, major technology companies, cable companies, and large hotel chains. There is much more to pornography than personal choice as it relates to sexual expression and personal choice. It is a global industry where the bodies of men, women and children are exploited for profit. It is a large network of sexual exploitation that deliberately recruits from shelters and foster homes. In other words they seek out the most vulnerable people to feed a supply chain that desperately requires a supply of fresh bodies due to the extent of the degradation and physical punishment that is associated with producing pornographic material.

According to studies, men watch pornography for several different reasons. Here are some of them:

It's safer than random sex: This reason should only apply to single men; however, in this age of infidelity it probably doesn't. Although society is a proponent of casual sex, there are some men who are just not into it and would rather wait until they are in a committed relationship. There is a fear of sexually transmitted diseases, awkward conversations the next morning, and hurt feelings. Men need to find some type of release while they are waiting for the right woman and they get that through pornography and masturbation. Men get the release they need, it eliminates the fear of rejection and performance anxiety and they have access to it whenever they want.

Visual stimulation: Men are visual creatures, they like looking at women they find appealing. They like watching their women during sex which is one of the reasons why they like to change positions. Watching porn leaves nothing to the imagination; men can just watch and enjoy watching.

Vicarious living: Pornographic scenes are not the norm, having sex in the middle of restaurants, sex on the mangers desk, sex with a desperate housewife when the husband is away. A lot of men wish that they had so much sexual freedom, when they are watching porn they can imagine that it's them carrying out the act.

It allows men to be selfish: At times, men enjoy masturbating more than sex because it allows them to focus completely on their own pleasure. When a man is having sex with a woman he wants to please her and in order to do so he has to be totally engaged in the act, reading her body language and making sure they don't peak too quickly. Pornography adds to the intensity of male fantasy.

Men like to strategize: Men like to plan what they are going to do and how they are going to do it before they do it. Watching porn gives them ideas about what positions they can carry out in the bedroom.

Is there a solution to this problem? It might be too late for this generation, but for the ones coming behind us it is essential that schools play a larger role in sex education. This should involve more than the physiological process of sex and how the male and female body works to produce babies. At present this is all that is being taught in schools. There needs to be more emphasis placed on the emotional connection to sex, passion, feelings and communication. It is clear that teaching teenagers about biological logistics simply isn't enough.

Young boys are spending so much time watching pornography that they are internalizing an unrealistic portrayal of sexual relationships. The education system should be responsible for injecting the truth about sex and sexuality into the minds of our young people to assist them in developing the emotional skills required to maintain a healthy relationship.

Pornography has been normalized and many men and women don't think there is anything wrong with watching it. However, it appears that the effects of an addiction to it are devastating.

Chapter 9: Addicted to Pornography

Addiction to pornography happens when the person watching it is unable to control whether or not they will engage in the behavior they are exposing themselves to. A porn addict watches porn as an act of compulsion regardless of the consequences they may face which include:

- An inability to form meaningful romantic, intimate and social relationships

- Intense feelings of shame, depression and isolation

- The breakdown of relationships with romantic partners, friends and family

- Hours and perhaps days wasted watching pornography

- A loss of interest in activities that do not involve pornography such as exercise, family, socializing, school and work

- Trouble at school or work for watching porn on a school or work computer

- Financial issues due to excessive spending to fuel their addiction

- Legal issues related to viewing illegal images

- Porn addiction combined with drug or alcohol addiction

- Physical injury as a result of excessive masturbation

- Sexual dysfunction in relationships including an inability to have an orgasm because they are not exposed to pornography. The inability to get or sustain an erection because they are not being exposed to pornography

The life of an addict spirals out of control because they are constantly chasing that first high. Addicts feel the need to keep using even though the effectiveness of the drug is no longer the same. The first time a drug is used the brain's reward receptors get accustomed to the feelings of pleasure that are associated with the drug. This experience sets up a vicious cycle of abuse as your brain is programmed to seek that first time high over and over again. The brain starts to associate use with the euphoric feeling it experienced when it was first introduced to the drug as opposed to the actual experience of using the drug.

One of the psychological effects of drugs and alcohol is that the more a person uses, they continuously need a higher dosage to achieve the same results. This is when addiction gets dangerous; attempting to reach peak effects by increasing the amount taken puts the addict at risk of damage to major organs and overdose.

Another reason why an addict chases the first high is that when they are not they are exposed to the effects of a severe low. This is due to the fact that the same reward receptors that have become so attached to being rewarded that they send a signal to the brain when they are not. It is this that causes the low.

Addiction is the same regardless of the focus, the same way drug addicts chase their first high is the same way porn addicts chase their first high.

In an attempt to experience the same feelings as when they were first exposed to pornography they start searching for more graphic images. This is often how child pornography is introduced. The addiction has spiraled out of control and they now get aroused by images that go against their moral values. This leads them to experience a massive amount of shame about what they are doing which leads to a stressful and secretive double life. For the majority of addicts, the stress is so intense that it affects their emotional and physical lives.

Causes

In the same way that a sex addict is not having sex primarily because of the pleasure associated with the act, the porn addict doesn't watch pornography primarily because of the sexual enjoyment attached to watching it. Instead, the addiction is viewed as a way of escape from unresolved trauma due to neglect or abuse, low self-esteem, anxiety, depression, stress and emotional discomfort. Alcoholics and drug addict's use for exactly the same reasons. Porn addicts don't want to feel, or at the very least they want to control what they are feeling.

Addiction triggers a pleasurable chemical response in the brain; this is fueled by the release of a neurotransmitter known as dopamine, and other biochemicals such as endorphins, serotonin, adrenaline, and oxytocin. As time goes on, porn addicts learn to abuse this natural reaction in the same way that drug addicts and alcoholics learn to abuse their drink or drug of choice. Their aim is to intentionally trigger the pleasure response associated with sexual fantasy and pornography. The addict uses the high to avoid feelings of anxiety, depression and other stressors.

Like any other addict, a porn addict likes to remain high for as long as possible. They are therefore more interested in using pornography to maintain their intense sexual fantasies as opposed to reaching orgasm. For a porn addict, having an orgasm terminates the high and quickly propels them back into the real world which is what they want to avoid. As a result, porn addicts can spend hours and maybe even days zoned out in a neurochemical bubble fantasizing about sexual activity and watching porn without engaging in sex or masturbation.

Porn Addiction Symptoms

Although statistics show that there are more men addicted to pornography than women, both sexes can become addicted to porn. The content of the porn is different with men preferring hardcore porn of purely sexualized images and women having a preference for erotica that has a hint of an emotional connection. Either way, the symptoms of porn addiction are the same and they typically include the following:

- Copious amounts of time spent watching pornography and searching for the right images that will cause arousal

- Progressively viewing more bizarre and more intense sexual content

- Continued use of porn despite making promises to others and self to stop watching it

- Keeping secrets, lying and covering up the severity of porn use

- Irritability or anger about when confronted with the extent and nature of porn use

- Escalation of porn use from viewing to interacting with people willing to engage in pornographic acts such as web cam, phone sex and visiting prostitutes

Risk Factors

There are many risks associated with porn addiction and they are no different to the risks associated with any other type of addiction. Research indicates that someone who was abused or neglected during childhood has a higher risk of becoming an addict. The younger a person is when first introduced to an addictive substance or starts to engage in addictive behavior the more at risk that person is to becoming an addict. Porn addiction stems from a combination of risk factors including poor parenting leading to an early exposure to pornography, environmental factors and genetic disposition.

Chapter 10: When Sexual Expression Breaks Down Marriages

Ten years into her marriage, Sarah began to wonder if her husband no longer had any interest in sex. "He started to go to bed later than me and when I questioned him about it he would make excuses." Explains the 43 year old. "So when he finally decided to talk to me about what was really going on, I started laughing when he said that he was a sex addict. Although that laughter was short lived when he began to reveal that he has had a string of short affairs and comes to bed late because he spends hours watching pornography. I felt as if my world had come to an end."

Paula Hall, the author of *"Sex Addiction: The Partner's Perspective"* states that sex addiction destroys couples faster than any other addiction. She states that when you are the partner sex addiction is personal because it has an effect on the most intimate element of your relationship in a way that alcohol or drug addiction isn't able to.

"I could of handled an addiction to gambling, alcohol or even drugs but I couldn't cope with sex addiction." Sarah confirms. Like the majority of partners, at first she didn't believe there was such thing as sex addiction because it just sounded like a weak excuse to have an affair. After doing the research and she finally started to believe in her husband's addiction, her friends didn't. They would look at her in despair, with a refusal to understand how sexual urges can become so strong that a man is unable to control them. This left her feeling alone and isolated.

To be fair on Sarah's friends there is a lot of debate as to whether sex addiction is actually a scientific term, but the field of addiction is quickly shifting, and there is more of an emphasis on the psychological symptoms of addiction as opposed to the substance. Sex addiction comes under the banner of actually engaging in sexual activity, using sex chat lines, paying for sex with prostitutes, masturbation and pornography.

There are many complex reasons surrounding sex addiction; however, according to Hall for the vast majority it is simply a matter of opportunity. The Western world is now structured in such a way that you can get anything you want anonymously and easily and then become addicted to it.

Traditionally, the majority of partners in a relationship with a sex addict have been treated as a co-dependent. To some extent the partner knew that what was taking place and through their failure to confront it were enabling it. This view is completely unfair, but it exists. The reality is that when most partners discover sex addiction they are in total shock and their self esteem is completely destroyed. For the most part, it isn't just about the sexually deviant behavior such as visiting a prostitute. What hurts the most is the fact that they have been living with someone for such a long period of time and they were not aware of this side of them. In general it is men who are exposed as sex addicts and they are typically loving husbands and fathers. Yet, they have committed such an abominable act right under the nose of the person they are supposed to love and cherish forever. At this point trust is broken and fixing it can seem impossible.

Many partners suffer from severe trauma after the discovery which leads to dissociation, rage, panic attacks, anxiety and depression. In Halls book one sassy businesswoman talks about how she no longer recognized herself after she found out about her husband's sex addiction. Something came out of her that she didn't know was possible. Hall believes that partners need just as much help as the sex addict when the truth is revealed and she addresses some self help techniques in her book. Because this is a relatively new area of psychotherapy, some therapists make the same assumptions as well meaning friends about sex addiction. They find it difficult to believe and so they work with the partner as if they are treating a victim of infidelity and there are so many more layers to it than that. You need to remember that there are some people who are not actually physically participating in sex outside of their relationship; they are using porn, sex chat lines and web cam.

Not only is Hall an author, she is also the owner of a therapeutic practice that recognizes the unique nature of a partners pain. Her business has grown tremendously simply because of her revelation knowledge into what a partner has to deal with psychologically. Sex addiction for the partner provokes feelings of insecurity, "He's not attracted to me" or "I will never be able to satisfy him," but the addiction isn't about having sex, it's about getting a dopamine fix. As soon as a partner is able to understand the nature of addiction they can then start the healing process.

Research has concluded that a third of partners looking for help remain in the relationship, a third move on, and a third stay trapped without getting the help that they need. The couples who are able to overcome it typically take a three pronged approach:

1. The addict seeks psychological help to determine the cause of the addiction. They are also provided with strategies to prevent relapse

2. The partner learns about addiction, they work on making the partner feel stable

again and discuss what they want for the future.

3. The couple work together to form boundaries in the relationship

While some addicts are able to overcome the addiction, it is important that the partner is able to recognize that they are going to be living with someone who is in lifelong recovery. Nobody is advising partners to remain in a dysfunctional relationship; for some partners leaving is the best decision for them. However, when they do leave, they must remember that they are going to need support to rebuild trust and reclaim their sexuality when they get into another relationship.

Sarah agrees. "My husband tried his best to gain control of his behavior through learning about the nature of sex addiction. The problem was that he wasn't as forth coming in dealing with the root cause of the problem. That meant that there was a high chance of him relapsing and I wasn't prepared to go through that again so I left. Once I had let go of the relationship I had to get help for myself or I would never have been able to move forward with my life.

Chapter 11: The Religious View of Sexual Expression

It appears that human beings don't know how to do anything right, hence the state of the world today. Everyone seems to have their own ideals, values and morals that nine times out of ten lead down the road to nothingness. I have decided to include the religious view of sexual expression simply because it's an opinion that a certain group of people strongly believe in. Whether it's right or wrong is debateable, but it is certainly interesting.

Christians believe that the person who created the human race (God) designed sex for marriage only and that the world, due to cultural influences has got the wrong idea about it.

Christian counselor Waylon refers to this problem as the "Pickle Principle." Waylon states that making pickles involves putting cucumbers into a solution of brine vinegar, water and spices. After the cucumber has been soaked in the brine for the right amount of time it changes into a pickle. The majority of the human race is like a pickle. We sit in the brine of a culture that has been saturated by sex, absorbing its values and beliefs and it conditions our thinking.

The brine that the world has been saturated in includes the belief that people have the right to satisfy their sexual urges by engaging in sex with whomever they please. The message delivered to the world through music, movies and TV is that there is nothing more pleasurable than sex, and every individual whether young or old can participate in it freely. Another element of the pickling process is that people are entitled to express themselves sexually in any way that they please and no one has got the right to give their opinion on what is right or wrong about this expression.

If the main aim of sex is for pleasure then human beings are simply objects of sexual gratification. The Christian perspective is that pleasure is the by product of sex in a relational context, and that relationship is marriage. The book that Christians learn about their beliefs is referred to as the Bible; they believe that the words in it are instructions from God about how to live on earth. The Bible teaches that sex binds two souls together, it has got so much power that the safest environment for it to take place is within the committed   covenant   of   the   marriage relationship.

God Invented Sex

Christians believe that the creator of mankind invented sex. He didn't only make it for the purpose of procreation but for it to be deeply satisfying and pleasurable. He designed the body parts of men and women to complement each other with hormones to initiate the desire for sex. Unlike animals, who are purely instinctive for the purpose of reproduction when it comes to their mating behavior, there are several purposes for human sexuality and all of them should stay within a marriage.

In a lifetime covenant of faithfulness between a married couple, we can enjoy and express God's two main purposes for sex: Intimacy and fruitfulness. When the first human beings Adam and Eve were created, they were given a command to "be fruitful and multiply" (Genesis 1:28). One of the purposes of sex is to create human beings. However, the concept of fruitfulness is not limited to having children. A mutually loving relationship between husband and wife can also produce personal and emotional fruitfulness where both parties support each other to become the best versions of themselves.

The other purpose of sex is for physical and emotional intimacy and this should only take place within a marriage. Eric Elder wrote a book entitled "What God Says About Sex." He describes how it is only safe to completely reveal yourself to a person once you are in the safety of a committed marriage. The fullest freedom and experience of sex can only be found in the marital bed. God commands us to be disciplined and self controlled in order to keep sex within this context.

Sex also builds a strong union between two people, husband and wife become one flesh and they are joined together through a shared life. From the Christian perspective sex is like solder that is used for the fusion of metal. Once two people are joined together there is a strong bond that holds the marriage and the family intact which is what God planned for our lives. Sex is also for the purpose of pleasure and it can be experienced in the safety of a loving marriage.

So What Does The Bible Really Say About Sex

Many non Christians believe that God has so many rules and regulations because he doesn't want us to have any fun, and since sex feels good, he doesn't want us to do it. This view is in direct contradiction to what the Bible says. From my studies, God doesn't seem to have a problem with us having as much sex as we want just as long as it takes place within the right environment and that's marriage. The Biblical view of sex and the world's view of sex are polar opposites, but if you dig a little deeper you will find that one makes more sense than the other whether you are religious or not.

The fact that God has instructed us to have sex within a marriage context means that any other form of sexual expression is forbidden, and not because God is some kind of cosmic kill joy but because He created us and He knows what's best for us. Christians refer to God as their Father, He is the one who created them, a loving parent knows what's best for their child. When a mother sees their toddler going to put their hand on the hot stove they immediately stop them from doing so and then tell them why they shouldn't touch it with the reason being that it's hot and it will burn you. God is no difference, He tells us to abstain from sex until marriage and if we choose to do it anyway there are consequences. Let's take a look at them.

The Consequences of Sexual Expression

Sexual freedom has been flaunted as the norm. In fact, it's common to be labeled as "weird" if you choose to remain a virgin until marriage. (This is especially true of men) Behind every Biblical command that appears negative there are two positive principles, one of them is for our protection and the other is for our provision. The person who created us has a plan for how we are to live our lives and He doesn't want us to do anything that will cause us pain. To illustrate this, let's look at the owner manual that comes with an automobile. Once I've bought the car I might decide that I want to change the oil once a year because it will save me time and money. However, the owner manual says that I should have an oil change every 5,000 miles. If I have any sense, I will trust that the person who created the car has better knowledge about how to care for it than I do. If I follow their advice instead of doing what I want to do I am sure it will save me money and grief from having to deal with the consequences.

If we look at this analogy from a Biblical perspective, yes it feels good to have sex with whoever we are attracted to but the "Owners manual (the Bible) doesn't agree. So who should we believe our cultural values or God? He created sex, but there are rules that we have to abide by, isn't it interesting that the majority of us are ok with abiding by the rules with everything else such as sports and driving. Can you imagine a basketball match without any rules? Can you imagine the roads without any rules? There would be complete anarchy and chaos. God has one rule for sex, and that is not to do it unless you are married, let's see what happens when it's broken.

Sexually Transmitted Diseases (STD)

Fifty years ago teenagers were warned about two sexually transmitted diseases, back then they were referred to as "venereal diseases," gonorrhoea and syphilis. What has sexual freedom given us? More than 50 STDs. According to the University of Maryland Medical Center, over 13 million Americans are affected by STDs each year and three of them are fatal:

- **Human Immunodeficiency Virus (HIV):** According to the Centers for Disease Control and Prevention (CDC) HIV destroys the cells required by the body to fight off infection and disease. It basically breaks down the immune system making you more susceptible to other serious illnesses such as acquired immunodeficiency syndrome (AIDS) and cancer, both of which are fatal.

AIDS is the last stage of HIV, by this point the immune system has become so weak that the sufferer becomes vulnerable to life threatening illnesses such as pneumonia and tuberculosis. Once diagnosed with pneumonia or tuberculosis, life expectancy is reduced to one year. There is no cure for HIV, the virus can only be controlled and treated.

- **Hepatitis B:** Although the majority of people were vaccinated against hepatitis B as children, there is still a risk of becoming infected. According to the CDC, Hepatitis B is a contagious disease of the liver; it is typically passed on through sexual conduct. If chronic hepatitis develops it leads to cirrhosis of the liver that can escalate into liver cancer, kidney failure, and diabetes.

- **Human Papillomavirus (HPV):** According to the National Cancer Institute HPV is an infection that belongs to a group of more than 200 other viruses and over 40 are spread through sexual contact. When HPV remains inside the body, it can cause cervical cancer and genital warts.

If an expectant mother suffers from gonorrhoea she can pass the condition on to her child as it passes through the birth canal. It can also cause eye infections in the baby, stillbirth and premature birth. I could go on but I think you get the point. The God that the Christians believe in says that the only way to protect yourself against sexually transmitted diseases is to have sex within the constraints of marriage only. How does our culture tell us to protect ourselves against STDs? By making sure you wear a condom and limiting the number of sexual partners you have. The majority of people who are sexually active know how unreliable condoms can be, they break and they slip off.

However, even if the condom stays on, the same sperm that gets a woman pregnant can get through a pinhole or a tiny tear in a condom. The virus that causes AIDS is approximately 300 to 400 times smaller than the semen. The same tiny tear to the AIDS virus looks like a train tunnel!

Cervical Cancer

According to leading British scientist Professor Julian Peto promiscuous teenage girls are at risk of developing cervical cancer later on in life. His research concludes that becoming sexually active at a young age and unprotected sex with multiple partners increases the risk of HPV which is the virus that causes cervical cancer. Professor Peto believes that the virus can stay in a woman's body which increases the risk of developing cervical cancer. In the United Kingdom 3,000 women are diagnosed every year and out of those 3,000 it kills 1,300 women.

The warning came when sexually transmitted diseases were at a ten year high among young people in England. It appears that a woman's sexual history can return to haunt her when she is in her 50's after being in a faithful marriage for years. Scientists have also warned that the STD Chlamydia has a strong link to cervical cancer.

Abortion

There is still an argument as to whether abortion is the killing of another human being, but whether it is or it isn't unwanted pregnancy is clearly a worldwide problem. According to the World Health Organization there are approximately 40-50 million abortions globally each year. In America almost half of all pregnancies were unintentional and 4 in 10 end in abortions. Some may argue that a woman has the right to do what she wants with her body, and it's her choice if she wants to give birth or not. However, there are also consequences to abortions both physically and emotionally, let's take a look:

Emotional side effects include the following:

- Anxiety

- Depression

- Eating disorders

- Suicidal thoughts

- Relationship issues

- Low self esteem

- Loneliness and isolation

- Shame

- Guilt

- Anger

- Regret

Physical side effects include the following:

- Organ damage

- Persistent or heavy bleeding

- Death

- Perforation of the uterus

- Scarring to the lining of the uterus

- Cervix damage

- Sepsis or infection

What Happens During Sex

In chapter 3 I talked about the feminist who claimed she liked having sex with multiple partners but got upset when they treated her like a sex object, well this section will explain why. When two people have sex, oxytocin is released in the brain; this hormone creates a bond between the two people. It sounds similar to the following verse in the Bible "For this reason a man shall leave his father and mother and be joined to his wife, and the two shall become one flesh, so then they are no longer two but one flesh." (Mark 10:7-8)

Dr Daniel Amen one of the most prominent figures in the area of neuropsychology states in his book "Change Your Brain Change Your Life," that the release of oxytocin creates limbic emotional bonding and this is the reason why casual relationships never work out. Two people might decide to have a one night stand, yet something is taking place in another realm that they had not planned. Whether they want it to happen or not, sex is producing an emotional bond between the couple. The woman often forms a deeper emotional attachment because she has a larger limbic system (the seat of our emotions) than men. She then ends up getting hurt. The emotional attachment formed during sex is the glue that holds people together in a relationship. Taking the conversation back to pornography, this is one of the reasons why it is so dangerous.

When a man watches pornography, masturbates and reaches orgasm the main hormone released is dopamine which is responsible for causing addiction due to the fact that it activates the reward center in the brain when a goal is accomplished. These neurological and hormonal consequences were designed to create a bond between the man and the object of his focus. God planned that this would be the woman he was married to; however, for the many men who engage in watching pornography it is the image on the screen. Pornography therefore enslaves the viewer to what he is looking at, hijacking the biological response that was intended to bond husband and wife.

Despite the fact that casual sex is so popular Dr Amen is even bold enough to state that theoretically speaking it isn't possible to have casual sex because of the emotional bond that has been created. This is why one night stands can become addictive, people develop a desire to have an emotional bond because of the chemical reaction that is taking place within the brain but they are not willing to settle down in a relationship.

Conclusion

It is clear that there is a problem with sexual expression. We live in a society with conflicting norms and values. Due to a lack of sexual education teenagers are confused about sexuality and the media is training adolescents to believe that their bodies are nothing but commodities to be bought and sold. Pornography has become an epidemic and children as young as ten are being exposed to graphic images which end up shaping their identity and further confusing them about their role in life.

As we have discussed the consequences of sexual freedom are fatal, safe sex is only as safe as playing Russian roulette with your life, one wrong "split" and its game over for you! Waiting until marriage sounds almost convincing until you factor in the chances of marrying someone with a porn addiction and having to deal with a partner who would rather have sex with a screen than with you. So what's the solution? I can't answer that question; however, what I can tell you is that there are people in the world who have made up in their mind that they are not going to conform to the ways of this world; they have got principles, values, morals and integrity. They live disciplined lives and they are intelligent enough to know that society and the culture that we live in has got it backwards and will not allow its influences to dictate how they choose to live. Weigh the pros and cons of living a life of sexual freedom and sexual expression and decide what voice are you going to listen to!

CPSIA information can be obtained
at www.ICGtesting.com
Printed in the USA
LVHW091129230122
709160LV00020B/178